Over 50 Fitness:

The Best Ways to Lose Weight As A Woman Over 50

AMY T. DAVID

2016 Copyright © AMY T. DAVID

All rights reserved. No part of this guide may be reproduced in any form without permission in writing from the publisher except in the case of brief quotations embodied in critical articles or reviews.

Legal & Disclaimer

The information contained in this book is not designed to replace or take the place of any form of medicine or professional medical advice. The information in this book has been provided for educational and entertainment purposes only.

The information contained in this book has been compiled from sources deemed reliable, and it is accurate to the best of the Author's knowledge; however, the Author cannot guarantee its accuracy and validity and cannot be held liable for any errors or omissions. Changes are periodically made to this book. You must consult your doctor or get professional medical advice before using any of the suggested remedies, techniques, or information in this book.

Upon using the information contained in this book, you agree to hold harmless the Author from and against any damages, costs, and expenses, including any legal fees potentially resulting from the application of any of the information provided by this guide. This disclaimer applies to any damages or injury caused by the use and application, whether directly or indirectly, of any advice or information presented, whether for breach of contract, tort, negligence, personal injury, criminal intent, or under any other cause of action. You agree to accept all risks of using the information presented inside this book. You need to consult a professional medical practitioner in order to ensure you are both able and healthy enough to participate in this program.

Table of Contents

Introduction	6
Chapter 1: How is Weight Loss For Women Over 50 Different?	8
Chapter 2: The Truth About Your Body Over 50: What You Can Change?	12
Chapter 3: Understanding Nutrition Over 50	18
Chapter 4: The Healthiest Foods For Your Body	23
Chapter 5: The Diet Plan	
Breakfast Options	30
Lunch Options	31
Dinner Options	33
Snack and Dessert Options	35
Chapter 6: Best Exercises For Women Over 50	37
Conclusions	41
Check Out Other Books	42

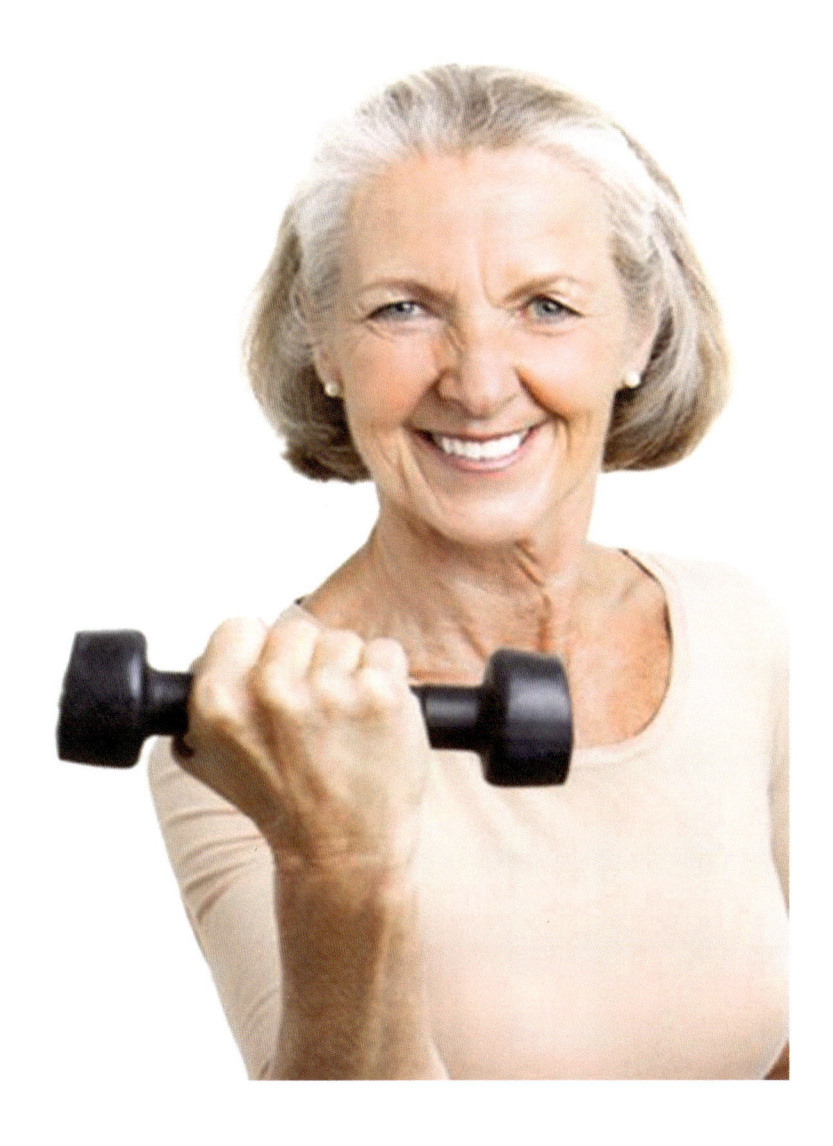

"And the beauty of a woman, with passing years only grows!"
— Audrey Hepburn

Introduction

When you get to be over 50 it can be more difficult to lose weight. You want to make sure that you're in good shape but, at the same time, you find yourself struggling. The truth is that a lot of people experience these problems. The biggest thing you can do is make sure that you're eating healthy and that you're exercising right, but when you get to be over 50 these things can actually change. You find yourself gaining weight without changing anything. That's the unfortunate truth about getting older. So what can you do?

This book is all about exactly that. We're going to help you understand what you need to do in order to lose weight as a woman over 50. You don't have to live with a weight that you don't like or with anything that you aren't completely happy about. You only get one life to live after all. Shouldn't you be able to enjoy every minute of it? You don't want to spend your life missing out on things because of your weight or because of your energy levels (which decrease as your weight goes up).

We're going to talk about some of the best ways that you can lose weight. We'll explain some great exercise programs and some of the best exercises that you can use to start losing some of that weight and toning up the body you do have. There are more methods than you will believe and each one of them is going to appeal to different people. If you want something more hardcore we have some of those, but we also have some lower intensity workouts for those who are just getting started or more interested in losing weight than bulking up.

Another important aspect is the diet. Your diet is going to influence the weight that you are able to gain or lose so of course we're going to go over some of the best things you can eat for your diet and what you need to do to cut some of the pounds. Dieting doesn't have to mean missing out on things that you enjoy. So take the time to read through our chapter on nutrition to find out what your body really needs and what it can do for you. Then make sure to read more about the diet that's going to help you get the body you've always wanted.

Chapter 1: How is Weight Loss For Women Over 50 Different?

When you're a little bit older it can be more difficult to lose weight. Unfortunately, that's also when you start putting on a little extra weight. So what can you do? Well there are actually quite a few ways that you can go about losing weight. You just have to understand that it's not going to be quite the same as when you were younger. You will have to put a little bit more work into it. But the great thing is you can still get your weight under control and you can still get yourself where you want to be.

Now, let's start with why you gain weight in the first place. When you get to be 50 your body typically goes through menopause. Now this can happen a little before 50 or just after 50, but it will strike you right about this time. Then you'll find yourself putting on at least a few extra pounds. Not necessarily because you're eating differently, but because your body just stops breaking it down the way that it used to. You want to make sure that you're prepared for this, but if you're not ... well then you want to be prepared to get rid of that weight.

Over 50 years old you, once you go through menopause, you are actually at higher risk of developing some pretty serious health conditions if you start putting on a lot of weight. You want to make sure that you're paying attention to this. Putting on weight at any age increases your risk of developing health problems like high blood pressure and even diabetes or heart attacks. Once you get older however, you're actually at higher risk for developing breast cancer. The worst thing is if you're gaining the weight actually during menopause and not just after.

So why do you gain so much weight when you get to be over 50 years old? You gain weight because most people start behaving differently. Once you start to get older you start to feel differently about your body and your body starts to react differently as well. You start to exercise a little less, maybe eat a little less healthy. But what's really hurting your body is that your metabolism and the way your body processes food will change as well. It's important to be prepared for these changes and to understand that your body needs more help than it did when you were younger.

Your food and exercise needs are going to change when you get to this age and that means you're going to need some big changes in your body. You need to make sure that you eat properly and that you're eating enough food as well. We'll talk in another chapter about the specifics of what you should be eating and why you need more or less of it. For now, suffice it to say that you're going to need to make a lot of changes to stay healthy.

If you were healthy when you were under 50 you'll have a better chance of staying healthy as you age. But remember it's going to get more difficult. You'll have a lot more muscle mass loss just because you start to get older and, unfortunately, you're also going to find yourself burning a lot less calories at all times of the day. When you're younger your body actually burns calories just by sitting and doing nothing. When you get older however … this is no longer going to happen. Your body won't be able to burn as many calories as you're simply sitting and doing nothing.

That means if you decide to do absolutely nothing different and you opt to just continue eating, drinking and exercising the same way you did before 50, you're actually going to gain weight. It doesn't matter if you continue your entire routine exactly the same down to the last tenth of a calorie. You will gain weight because your body just doesn't burn those calories the same way that it used to. It's not fair, but it's something you definitely need to start thinking about and start working on.

So, unfortunately, as you get older, you're going to gain more weight and you're going to lose more muscle mass. This is going to result in more difficulty for you and it's going to result in more trouble getting rid of that excess weight and putting that muscle mass back where you need it to be. So how are you going to go about all of this? Well the rest of this book is going to talk about exactly that. We're going to give you some eating tips as well as some exercise routines that work best for women over 50 years who are looking to get in better shape.

Being in the best shape of your life does not need to happen when you're in your 20's. You can get back to that great shape again. All you need to do is make sure that you are putting your best foot forward and making strides towards what you want. Understand that it is possible. No matter what people may tell you, it is most definitely possible to get in better shape when you get older. You will be amazed at how great you look and feel and, once you start getting into great shape you're going to always want to be that way.

Take control of your life after 50. Don't let anyone tell you that you can't enjoy yourself or that you're going to have to settle for not looking as good as you want. Follow these fab over 50 tips and you're going to be happy that you started getting older. These can be the best years of your life if you just let them be. All it takes is some effort, some exercise and a new diet (but a good diet) and you'll be better off than ever before. You'll be the envy of all your friends.

Chapter 2: The Truth About Your Body Over 50: What You Can Change?

If you ask anyone their honest answer they will tell you that there is something about their body that they would like to change. Some have many things they'd like to change; some have only one or two. But everyone has something that they aren't 100% happy with. So what's the one thing that you would change about yourself if you could? What do you wish you could do differently with your body to make yourself feel better, look better or just *be* better? No doubt you can think of a couple things even if you don't admit it out loud.

When you start to get older you may start to feel more comfortable with your body but, at the same time, you start to notice even more problems. You start to develop wrinkles. You get a little more weight around your midsection. You get some saggy skin on your face. All of these things can start to make you even more self-conscious, just when you finally started to feel comfortable in your own skin. So what can you do about it? Well you can actually do quite a bit if you're willing to put in the work.

Now the first thing you can do is take care of yourself. We'll talk about the specifics of what to eat or drink and also what you should be doing as far as exercise. But for right now you should know that these things are going to play a big part in how you feel about yourself and what you are able to accomplish. Getting older means a lot of things about your lifestyle are going to change, from your energy levels to your hunger levels to how much exercise you really want to do in a given day.

There are plenty of other ways to take care of yourself however many of which are physical:

- Get Sleep – Now when you were younger you may have stayed out all night partying, drinking or even just watching movies with some friends. When you start to get older however, that kind of thing just isn't going to cut it anymore. You need to make sure you're getting enough sleep every night and that's going to mean at least 8 hours. The more sleep you get the better you're going to feel about yourself and the better you're going to do when it comes to the exercise you need to lose weight.

- Take Some Quiet Time – Now that your children are older or out of the house you have some time to take for yourself. Just relax and figure out what you want to do. You might read or meditate or pray. It's entirely up to you what you want and this is your time. Don't let anyone interfere with it (including you). That means you want to get up every morning with enough time for this ritual. It's going to help you feel calmer and more prepared to face the day, even though you'll get a little later start.

- Get Screenings – When you start to get older is when you're more at risk for different diseases. Anything from heart disease to cancer can start to pop up as you get older. That means it's time to start going to the doctor more regularly and get screened for any of those diseases. The last thing you want is to miss some appointments and find out later you have a serious disease. Most diseases can be treated if they are caught early enough so make sure you're catching them as quickly as possible.

- Get Bone Density Scans – Your bones will start to get a little weaker as you get older as well. The less calcium you get in your daily diet the worse off you're going to be. You want to talk with your doctor to find out the optimum level of calcium for you but for most people it's at least 1,200 milligrams. If you're not getting at least this much naturally through dairy products you may want to consider a supplement that's going to get you the levels you need. You definitely don't want to break a bone when you get older because it's going to take a lot longer to heal.

- Eat a Color Spectrum – The entire rainbow of foods is great for your body and it's something you will want to keep eating as you get older especially. After all, being over 50 can result in less vitamins and minerals in your body. You want to make sure that you are getting all of the things that you need because it's going to keep you healthier, something that also gets more important as you continue to age. So make sure you're getting plenty of different colors as you eat your meals every day. Those vitamins and minerals will help you feel better and look better.

- Do Some Aerobics – Aerobics, which we'll talk about later, are extremely important for your overall health. They're great for women over 50 because they actually require a lot less stress on your body. As a result, you start to get in better shape and you start to have a little fun at the same time. So make sure that you find a class and get involved. You're definitely going to be glad that you did once you realize that you're losing more weight than you were before. It's about flexibility, slow movements and enjoying yourself with friends after all.

- Drink Responsibly – No doubt you've heard this one before but it becomes even more important when you're older. Your body just won't hold alcohol the way that it did when you were younger so you have to be careful. You need to make sure that you're drinking only small amounts when you do drink (and don't do it as often as you used to either). This is going to ensure that you don't overdo it and that you are able to keep yourself healthy. After all, if you drink too much it can cause a number of additional health problems.

Another way to take care of yourself is to improve your mental health. By having some fun you can actually improve your mental health, something that can also start to decline as you get older. The problem is that most people start to feel upset, depressed or even angry when they get older. This makes it more difficult for them to enjoy their lives and it can even lead to diseases and premature death. You want to make sure that you're enjoying yourself by getting out there and participating in hobbies or activities that you really like.

- Enjoy Yourself – Make sure that you're having some fun as you get older. You can find a new friend, join a new class, or just go out with your partner or your family more often. You'll be able to have some fun and that's going to help you feel even better about yourself as well. You'll be surprised how great it is to just get out of the house once in a while. The more often you do it the better you're going to feel and the less risk you will have of developing health problems.

- Be Creative – Find something that you like to use to express yourself. That could be art, gardening, cooking or anything at all. As long as you enjoy it you're going to be able to improve your entire life. After all, what you may not realize is happiness is going to release endorphins in your brain. Those endorphins are going to help you feel better throughout the entire day. The more you release the longer and the better you're going to feel good about yourself. So what do you have to lose?

- Keep Your Mind Turned On – What you want to do is make sure that you're getting plenty of exercise, in your brain as well as your body. So make sure that you're exercising your mind by making yourself think. You can do this with brain teasers, word puzzle like crosswords or number puzzles. Just make sure that you're taking a little time each day to make your mind work for itself. Staying in the best shape of your life is not just about exercising to lose weight. You need to stay mentally sharp at the same time or you're just going to end up missing out on the great benefits that you were hoping to get from the extra exercise. There are all different ways to exercise your mind so try out a few different types of puzzle books and you'll find the right one for yourself in no time.

Chapter 3: Understanding Nutrition Over 50

Nutrition over 50 is different from nutrition for those who are under 50. The truth is your body has different needs than others and it has different needs than men as well. You need to make sure that you are following a nutrition and exercise plan that is intended for women and intended specifically for women over 50 because you could end up injuring yourself if you aren't careful.

If you're over 50 you need to make sure that you get plenty of calories each day. Of course, you actually want to eat a little less calories per day than someone under 50 because, if you remember, your body is going to burn less calories when it's resting than it would at any other time of your life. You want to cut down a little so you don't have to worry too much about exercising just to maintain your weight. What you want to do is exercise to lose weight.

So how many calories should you have in a given day? Well you should actually have about 1,600 to 2,200 calories in a single day (to maintain your weight). Remember this is going to account for everything that you eat (including meals and snacks) as well as everything that you drink over the course of a day. You should try to stick as close to these numbers as you can (at least once you talk to your doctor). Remember that your doctor knows your health the best. They will be able to tell you the best amount of calories for you to eat and remain healthy.

Now if you're looking to lose weight you're going to need to cut down on you calorie intake just a little. You don't want to cut too many calories too quickly because it could result in illness or it could be too little for your body to handle. Talking with your doctor will help you come up with your ideal number, but for most women it's going to be right around 1,200 calories, enough to keep you going throughout the day but not too much to make you pack on the pounds.

Keep in mind, if you're looking to lose weight you're going to need to eat the right types of foods rather than just eating 1,200 calories. We'll talk more about some of those 'right foods' in the next chapter when we go over some more about our diet plan but for now make sure that you're eating a little from every one of the food groups (a little less from the sugar and junk food category) but the more you get from each category the better off you're going to be and the better you're going to feel as well.

So what should you be eating? Well first you should make sure you're getting plenty of fiber. When you get older this becomes even more important because it helps you slow the absorption of glucose and it also helps to keep your cholesterol levels down, something you may otherwise have some problems with as you start to get older. More fiber will also be great for your diet because it helps you to stay full much longer. You won't eat as much and, as a result, you'll be able to lose even more weight. You should actually be getting at least 21 grams of fiber every day if you're over 50 years old.

Protein is another important thing for your diet and especially when you're a little older. The reason? Protein also helps you stay full a lot longer and it also helps you improve your strength and muscle mass. You'll be able to eat less but, at the same time, you won't be losing out on the muscle tone that would normally drop with a lower calorie diet. If you eat more protein you'll also feel better prepared to face the day. The ideal amount is about 0.68 grams per single pound.

Next, calcium. Nearly everyone has heard about this and knows that as you get older you start to have more difficulty with your bones. It happens because you're not getting enough calcium and, therefore, your body starts to take the calcium that it needs from your bones, which then get weaker. The weaker your bones get the more prone you are to breaking them and that can cause you a lot of pain and a lot of additional health problems. That's because broken bones take a lot longer to heal if you're older.

Of course, you want to make sure that you get plenty of antioxidants as well. These are going to help you fight off diseases, which can be even more dangerous if you're a little older. When you eat foods that are high in antioxidants you're going to help build up your immune system and you're going to be able to continue on with the rest of your life the way you want. After all, getting sick is definitely going to hurt your ability to carry on with your diet plan or your exercise plan or just having fun.

Some foods you need to make sure that you avoid are salt and fats (but only in certain ways). You want to make sure you aren't getting too much sodium in your diet because it can increase your blood pressure and lead to health problems such as heart disease or high cholesterol. Each of these increases your chances of cancers and other more serious diseases. The more sodium you take in the worse it's going to be for you. By decreasing the amount of sodium that you take in you'll be able to eat better and feel better at the same time.

Fats are a food to cut down on but they are not something you want to cut out entirely. That's because fats are actually good for you in a number of different ways. You just need to make sure that you're getting the right ones. Some of the 'wrong ones' are trans fats and saturated fats. Now you don't want to cut them out entirely, at least not the saturated fats. What you want to do is decrease the amount you're taking in so you don't end up with clogged arteries or a heart attack, which are both possible if you eat too much of these bad fats.

The fats that you do want are monounsaturated and polyunsaturated fats. They are going to keep you healthier and they are also going to ensure that you get good cholesterol. These fats are actually responsible for decreasing your risk of heart disease (contrary to what most people believe). You want to increase the amount of these fats you're eating (within reason of course) so that you get these benefits. Of course, as with anything, too much of this is going to result in additional health problems so make sure you're not eating a lot of fats of any type.

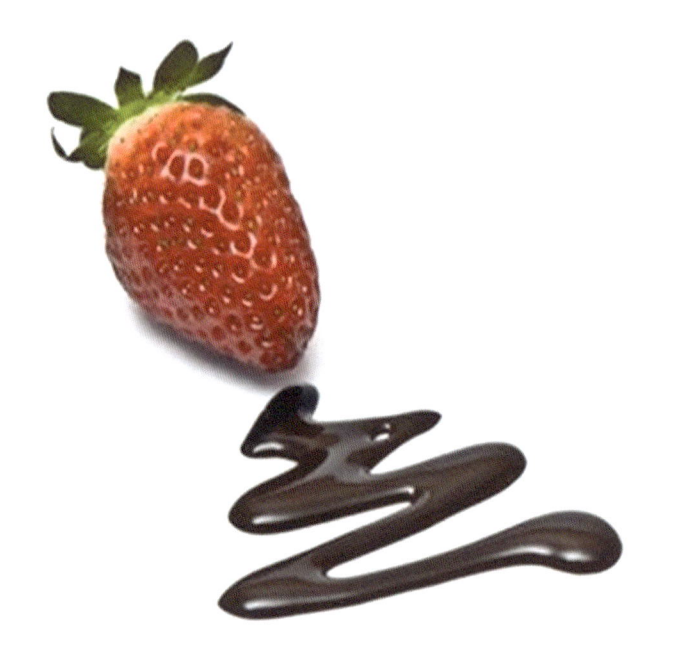

Chapter 4: The Healthiest Foods For Your Body

When you get to be 50 and over your body starts to change. As we've already mentioned a few times it starts to be even more important that you eat healthy and you watch your food intake. In this chapter we're going to talk about some of the most important foods that you should be eating as you get older. These foods are going to improve your overall health and keep you feeling better and actually acting better as well. You'll get more energy and your entire immune system and body will get a boost, resulting in less illness when it comes to everything from the common cold to cancer.

There are superfoods for every age group and for men and women alike. But the foods that you really want to eat when you're less than 50 years old are entirely different from the foods that are great for you over 50 (well not entirely but some are different). That means you want to make sure you're eating the right foods and the right quantities of them as well. This is going to require a little bit of change to your diet (possibly), but it's going to all be worth it when you get the body you've always wanted.

Superfoods are named the way they are because they have amazing benefits in a variety of different areas. Each superfood has more of some vitamin or mineral than nearly any other food and usually they have high levels of several different foods all at the same time. It's all about getting as much as you can from as few sources as possible. That way you don't have to spend all your time coming up with complicated meal plans and you can focus on more important things in your life.

1. Apples – Apples, with all the fiber that's in each one, are excellent over 50 because they help you decrease the levels of glucose in your body. Glucose is the sugar that your body needs in order to function, but too much glucose can actually cause problems and may result in heart disease, stroke or even kidney disease. But apples actually contain even more than fiber, they contain a lot of potassium, antioxidants and Vitamin C as well.

2. Asparagus – With a lot of extra lycopene, asparagus actually reduces your risk of prostate cancer. Anything that can reduce a cancer risk is definitely important to add in your diet. Plus, these veggies contain Vitamin A, fiber, protein and iron. So you're going to get quite a few all-around benefits. They relate to your eye and heart health as well as helping to improve your immune system. Just by including a little asparagus in your diet you're going to get all of these things plus reduction in bad cholesterol levels and more. And you don't need to eat a lot to do it.

3. Blueberries – Excellent for anyone, at any age, blueberries have a lot of fiber just like apples. But, on top of the high levels of fiber, blueberries also have a lot of Vitamin C and Vitamin K. These vitamins are going to help protect your heart and reduce your risk of osteoporosis. As you get older these can become extremely important concerns and that means you want to reduce your risk of them as much as possible. If eating blueberries is going to do it wouldn't you think twice about adding them to your diet?

4. Broccoli – This is probably one of the best vegetables that you could possibly eat because it has a lot of different vitamins and minerals. You're going to get not only a lot of fiber but plenty of antioxidants, Vitamin A, Vitamin B9, Vitamin C and Vitamin K. Each of these together is going to improve your entire body from your eyes and bones to your red blood cells, immune system and tissues. So if you've been avoiding broccoli for years it's definitely time to start eating it more often. You'll find plenty of ways to make it taste great and you'll be happy with the results it gives you too.

5. Butternut Squash – Filled with something called beta-carotene, butternut squash is excellent for adding fiber as well as improving cholesterol in your diet. The beta-carotene is actually able to improve your eye health, something that tends to decrease as you get a little older. It also helps to regulate your blood sugar so you reduce your risk of heart disease and stroke. With lower cholesterol levels you actually get a two-pronged attack on these two dangerous health conditions, because you're going to have a much stronger heart and body.

6. Dark Chocolate – Who needs convincing to add dark chocolate to their diet? I can bet most people are more than happy to eat a little more of this right? Well what you may not have known is that dark chocolate is actually good for you. The darker the chocolate you choose the better off you're going to be because the darker chocolate has a higher level of antioxidants, which help to keep you healthier by reducing your

change of clogged arteries. It will also reduce your blood pressure and reduce the risk of stroke. It's actually been found to reduce your risk by 20%.

7. Coffee – People who drink healthy are less likely to die by some of the most common methods affecting women over 50: heart and respiratory disease, stroke, diabetes, and accidents. It can even help to reduce your risk of developing breast cancer and Alzheimer's. If you drink more coffee during your 50's you will actually decrease your rate of developing Alzheimer's by 65%. Who wouldn't want that? Alzheimer's can be a really awful disease for those who suffer from it and for their families as well. If you can reduce your risk by that much wouldn't you want to take the initiative and do it? And with something you enjoy anyway.

8. Greek Yogurt – With almost twice as much protein as traditional American yogurt, Greek yogurt will give you less sugar, less carbs, less salt and a who much of probiotics. These are going to help improve your digestion and make it much easier for you to keep your body functioning the way that it should. You won't have to worry about your digestive tract because the probiotics are going to improve the way that your body breaks down food and gets rid of the things it doesn't need. Make sure to go with low fat versions that also have less saturated fats.

9. Pears – Another fruit that is full of fiber, pears are going to help you eat less because you'll feel full much faster. You'll also reduce your risk of diabetes and

colon cancer. Included in this fruit is a whole slew of different vitamins and minerals, including Vitamin C, folic acid, antioxidants and potassium, all of which combine to improve your immune system and help you stay healthy longer. You won't have to worry about digestion and you will be able to decrease your risk of developing osteoporosis, a common, but unfavorable condition among women as they start to get older.

10. Green Kale – Kale is one food that's going to revolutionize your diet because it's just so good for you. It has omega 3 fatty acids (which are the very best fats that you could have in your diet) as well as Vitamin K, fiber, calcium and lutein. That means you're going to get benefits to blood clotting, your bones and your eyes. The best part is you can eat it absolutely any way that you want. That means you can have it cooked or raw and you're going to get the same benefits. Not many foods can say that.

11. Fava Beans – These beans have fiber, folate, thiamin, riboflavin, manganese, iron and potassium. All of these are going to help you feel full much longer but they are also going to improve your immune system and your nervous system, keeping you from getting sick as frequently. If you're interested in keeping that healthy glow to your skin you're also going to want these beans because they can impact the way that your skin looks. As you get older you start to get dryness in your skin, but if you take the time to add some of these beans to your diet you won't have to worry as much.

12. Oatmeal – Loaded with fiber, protein, iron and more, oatmeal has very little fat and provides a simple cholesterol lowering formula. It helps your entire body and actually has a very low calorie count. Of course, you need to make sure you're eating real oats with very little additives. If you use instant oatmeal or you add a lot of extra ingredients you're not going to get as many benefits with oatmeal as you might think. What's great though is you can easily get a small canister of regular oats and make your own oatmeal in the morning quite fast.

13. Olive Oil – This is a great cooking oil if you're over 50 because it has a lot of monounsaturated fats, a fat that is healthier for your body. It helps reduce your risk of heart disease and even reduces your cholesterol. You'll even be able to reduce your insulin levels and balance out glucose. Want even more reasons to include it in your diet? It has high levels of Vitamin K, Vitamin E and more. So you'll get improved blood clotting and more red blood cells, which are essential to keeping your overall body much healthier.

14. Salmon – Possibly one of the best (and most certainly one of the most well-known) sources of Omega-3 fatty acids, salmon will help to reduce your risk of a heart attack and other heart problems as well. It even reduces your blood pressure, resulting in less risk of heart disease, stroke and more. If you have the choice make sure to choose wild-caught salmon which generally contains more of the omega 3 acids and less of some potentially harmful chemicals. You want all the benefits

you can get and when you start getting older you really want those acids to reduce your risk of serious conditions.

15. Quinoa – This grain is used by a number of vegetarians and vegans as well as those with gluten sensitivities. It is full of protein, antioxidants, Vitamin B2, magnesium, copper, phosphorous, fiber and iron, which means you get benefits to your entire body. You'll also get plenty of protein, which helps you to stay full much longer without reducing any muscle tone. If you're looking to get rid of some of the grains and pastas in your diet this is a healthy alternative. (Of course, you don't want to entirely get rid of grains because you want the fiber from them as well.)

Chapter 5: The Diet Plan

So now that you've seen some of the healthy foods that you should be eating you're probably wondering how you should be doing it. Well there are plenty of great meal plans out there for women who are over 50 but if you're trying to lose weight it's even more important to stick with the healthiest of those foods and keep your calorie count down. So how are you going to do that? Well you want to work with some of the healthy foods we talked about in the last chapter. Those are going to get you some weight loss benefits as well as some all-around health benefits.

Breakfast Options

Oatmeal With Blueberries
1 Cup Oatmeal (not instant)
¼ Cup Blueberries (fresh)

Mix together and enjoy for a low calorie breakfast that is also extremely healthy.

Quinoa With Vanilla and Blueberries
1 Cup Quinoa
1 Tablespoon Vanilla
2 Cups Fresh Blueberries
1 Tablespoon Coconut Oil
½ Teaspoon Cinnamon
2 Cups Water

Preheat your oven to 400 degrees Fahrenheit and combine quinoa, water and vanilla. Bring the mixture to a boil and then simmer for approximately 15 minutes or until all the water is absorbed. Bake blueberries with coconut oil and cinnamon on a parchment lined baking sheet for 15 minutes. Toss into quinoa and enjoy.

Yogurt Parfait
1 Cup Greek Yogurt
¼ Cup Blueberries (or to taste)
Other Fruit to Taste
Shaved Almonds

Layer half the yogurt and then all of one fruit. Top with rest of Greek yogurt and more fruit then with shaved almonds.

Lunch Options

Pear and Spinach Sandwich
2 Pears, cored, seeded, peeled and cut into ½" slices
2 Teaspoons Olive Oil
1 Teaspoon Lemon Juice
1 Cup Spinach
4 Slices Wheat Bread

Preheat your oven to 400 degree Fahrenheit then combine canola oil and lemon juice in a bowl. Toss together with pears and then place pears on a cookie sheet to roast for 20 minutes. They should be tender to the touch. Next, toast bread and top with pears and spinach.

Veggie Pesto Salad
8 Slices Wheat Bread
¼ Cup Low-Fat Shredded Mozzarella
2 Roma Tomatoes, sliced thin
1 Cup Arugula
¼ Cup Pesto

Toast bread until golden brown then add 1 tablespoon of mozzarella. Toast until the cheese melts then top with pesto, tomatoes and arugula.

Chicken Noodle Soup
1 Tablespoon Olive Oil
2 Carrots, Chopped
3 Celery Stalks, Trimmed and Diced
1 White Onion, Diced
4 Cups Chicken Stock
1 Teaspoon each Black Pepper, Garlic Powder & Dill Weed
1 Rotisserie Style Chicken
1 Cup Wheat Egg Noodles

In a 3 quart or larger pot, heat olive oil over medium-high heat. Add vegetables and sauté approximately 4 minutes. Disassemble the chicken, removing the skin and taking as much meat as possible from all bones.
Add your chicken stock and seasonings to the mixture in the pot and simmer over medium heat for approximately 5 minutes. Add half the chicken skin and 1 cup of meat with noodles to simmer for approximately 10 minutes. A foam should appear which you can remove along with the skin.

Dinner Options

Stuffed Chicken Breast
4 Boneless, Skinless Chicken Breasts
¼ Cup Each Crumbled Feta Cheese, Sun-Dried Tomatoes & Pitted Kalamata Olives
1 Tablespoon Each Chopped Fresh Dill and Parsley
2 Scallions
2 Tablespoons Olive Oil

Preheat your oven to 375 degrees Fahrenheit and season the chicken breasts with salt and pepper. Cut a slit in each side to create a small pocket that can be mixed with the feta mixture (to be made next).
Mix all ingredients (reserve 1 tablespoon olive oil) and stuff into chicken breasts. Seal the sides shut and sear in remaining olive oil until brown. Line a baking sheet with parchment paper and bake for an additional 12 minutes or until cooked completely. Make sure to let the chicken rest before you serve it.

Spicy Chili
1 Pound Ground Beef
1 Yellow Onion, Diced
2 Cloves Garlic, Minced
1 Can Each Kidney Beans, Black Beans, Fire-Roasted Tomatoes and Tomato Paste
2 Tablespoons Chili Powder
½ Teaspoon Each Black and Red Pepper Flakes
1 ½ Cups Water

Cook the ground beef with the onions and garlic in a large skillet. Make sure that most of the pink is gone from the meat and break up carefully. Drain fat and add (with all other ingredients) to slow cooker. Then simply cook for about 6-8 hours on low.

Asian Style Meatballs
1 Pound Ground Chicken
1 Egg
½ Cup Each Whole Wheat Bread Crumbs and Green Onions
1 Tablespoon Each Red Pepper Flakes and Sesame Seeds
2 Teaspoons Each Garlic Powder, Fresh Ginger and Cilantro
¾ Teaspoon Salt
3 Tablespoons Each Honey, Cider Vinegar and Tamari

Preheat your oven to 350 degrees Fahrenheit and mix the chicken, egg, bread crumbs, red pepper flakes, green onions, garlic powder and salt in a bowl. Allow breadcrumbs to expand slightly by letting the mixture sit for at least 15 minutes and roll into balls.
Line a baking sheet with parchment paper and allow to bake for approximately 22 minutes. Next, transfer them to a large skillet and drizzle with mixture of honey, vinegar and tamari. Cover the skillet and cook over medium heat, stirring every 2 minutes. Skillet should steam when done. Top with sesame seeds and cilantro.

Snack and Dessert Options

Strawberry Fruit Leather
4 Cups Strawberries

Preheat your oven to 150 degrees Fahrenheit and line with parchment paper. Process your strawberries in a food processor or blender until pureed. Pour onto baking sheet and cook for approximately 8 hours to reach desired doneness. Make sure to keep from getting too hard (should be tacky) so you have a chewy leather strip. Wait until they cool and cut into pieces.

Squash Fries and Yogurt Dip
1 Large Squash, Cut into ¼" Half Moons, Seeds Removed
2 Tablespoons Olive Oil
½ Teaspoon Salt
¾ Cup Greek Yogurt
1 Teaspoon Sriracha

Preheat your oven to 375 degrees Fahrenheit and line your baking sheet with aluminum foil. Toss squash with olive oil and lay out on baking sheet. Sprinkle some salt over the top to taste and bake for 20 minutes. Flip over each piece and bake another 25 minutes.
Increase oven to 500 degrees Fahrenheit and bake for 5 minutes, should be crispy.
Mix Greek yogurt with sriracha to form a dip for the fries.

Cucumber Tofu Rolls
1 Block Tofu, Extra Firm
1 Tablespoon Each Olive Oil and Fresh Ginger, Minced
2 Tablespoons Vinaigrette Dressing
½ Teaspoon Ground Cumin
1 Cucumber

Put the oil into a pan on a low-medium heat. Drain the tofu to get all excess liquid out and cut into 1/8" slices on the short side. Cut twice down the long side to form three rows of squares, approximately 36 total. Cook the tofu in the pan for about 15-20 minutes to brown and the flip to brown the other side.

Allow the tofu to cool while you slice the cucumber into 1/8" thick slices with a mandolin. Lay the slice on the cutting board, stack four pieces of tofu on top at one end and roll tightly. Use a toothpick to hold in place.

Chapter 6: Best Exercises For Women Over 50

When you start getting a little older you still want to make sure that you aren't pushing yourself too much when it comes to exercise. On the other hand, you want to make sure that you're getting plenty of it so that you can stay in the best shape of your life.

Aerobics are actually the best way that you can go about losing weight through exercise. They don't require a lot of strain on your body and they also help you burn a lot of calories at the same time. These types of exercise are actually quite common as well swimming, biking, walking, jogging and even dancing will help you get an excellent workout, without having to learn a new skill.

Of course, if you really want to get the best workout of your life you will want to try some new things. Take a new dance class, sign up for Pilates or just get out there jogging. If you get a group going you'll have even more fun and you'll be able to get a better workout because you're actually enjoying yourself. If you're able to talk while you exercise you're doing it right. You want a comfortable pace for at least 20 minutes 3 or more times each week to get the best results.

If you're looking for a little more specifics on your exercise program then try out these exercises:

3 Sets of 15 Squats
Squats are going to require some flexibility and they will require a lot of strength in your legs and abs as well. You need to spread your feet out wider than shoulder width (but not too much wider). Bring your arms straight out in front of you and push down with your heels into the ground as you lower your butt toward the ground.
You'll look like you're sitting on an invisible chair if you're doing it properly. Your thighs should be parallel to the ground with your knees bent at a 90 degree angle. Hold the position for a moment and then slowly rise back to a standing position.
If you want to add a little strength to the exercise you can add in some dumbbells to increase the weight and make it a little more difficult.

3 Sets of 1 Minute Planks
These are going to be a lot more difficult than you might think. What you want to do is lay down on your stomach with your elbows under your shoulders and your palms flat on the floor. Your toes should be pressed into the floor as well. Push yourself up with your hands and your abs so your body forms a 45 degree angle, from your toes through your head, with the floor. Your arms should form a 90 degree angle from your shoulders down to your hands, also with the floor. Hold this position for 1 minute and lower yourself to the ground before repeating.

3 Sets of 5 Pushups
Start with a plank formation, toes into the ground, hands under your shoulders and elbows near your sides. Push yourself up with your hands like you did for your plank but hold for a moment before slowly lowering yourself back down.

This process is different because you don't have to hold the plank at the top. Instead, you're just going to slowly rise yourself up and then slowly sink yourself back down. It's a much slower process.

Make sure you raise and lower your body slowly so you aren't wrenching anything and so you get the best results.

3 Sets of 15 Bicep Curls
Stand up tall with your feet shoulder width apart for balance. You won't actually need to use your legs for anything other than the balance.

Take weights that are slightly heavy (if you're looking to build muscle mass you will want heavier weights however for fat loss you will want only slightly heavy weights). Don't push yourself too hard.

Hold the weights down at your sides with the weights perpendicular to your feet. You want to make sure your knees aren't locked as this can cause you to pass out if you are not careful.

Bring the weights up toward your shoulders but do not bring them all the way up. The bicep is the muscle in the front of your arm. When you bring your weights up about halfway to your shoulders you are engaging the biceps. When you bring them all the way up you are engaging the shoulders. You want to work the biceps for this exercise so make sure you don't pull the weights up to far.

Make sure you also move slowly. Moving too quickly could damage the biceps or cause injury to you. The more reps you do the more fat you're going to lose. If you use heavy weights with a small number of repetitions you are going to increase your muscle mass rather than reducing the fat.

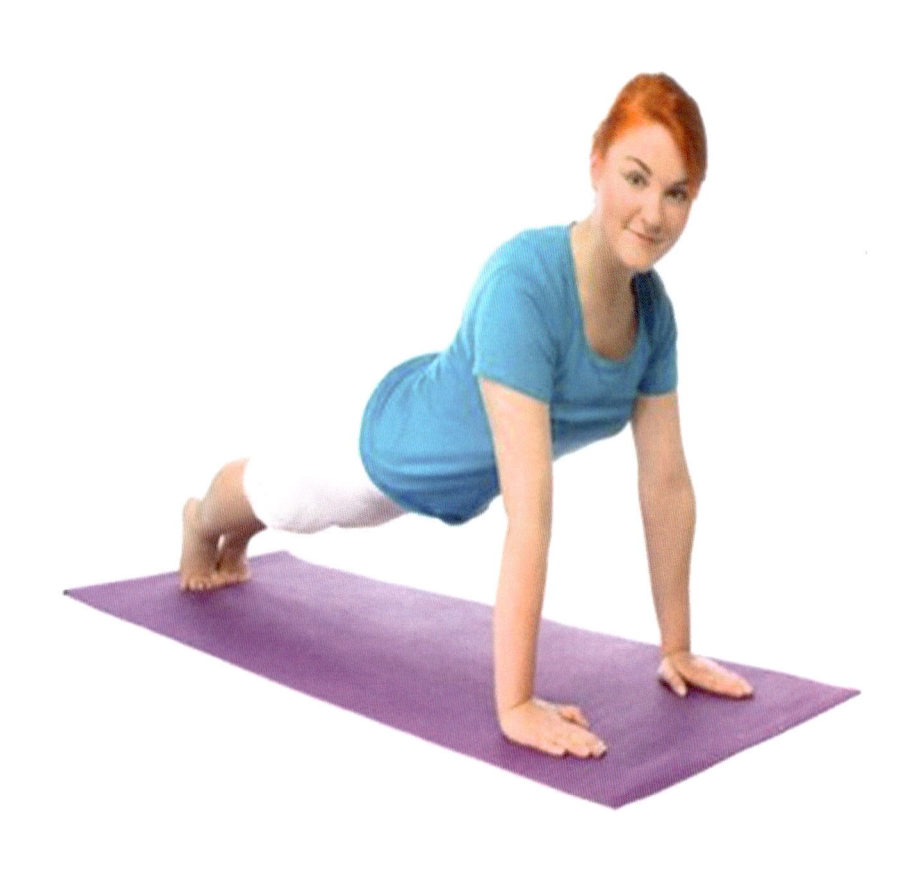

Conclusion

Ageing is inevitable; however, giving up the things that you enjoyed is not. Now, with a proper understanding of how weight loss is different for women over 50, you need to start eating healthy and exercising right. Women are like a fine wine. They only grow better with age.

So are you ready to lose some weight? Hopefully this book has been a big help to you. We've helped you to see some of the most important facts about weight loss and the ways that you're going to improve your entire life. It's all about helping your feel better and helping yourself to actually be better. You do not have to give up on all the things you want out of your life just because you're starting to get older. All you need to do is spend some time and effort on yourself.

When you take the time to get out there and start not only exercising but eating right and taking care of your entire body, you're going to start getting better at everything. You're going to feel better mentally and physically and emotionally as well. It's going to make you a better friend, a better partner, a better parent. You're going to be an all-around better you because you're going to feel like yourself, even though you're getting older. Don't let anything slow you down. This is your life to live and it's time that you do just that.

-- Amy T. David

Check Out Other Books in Amazon

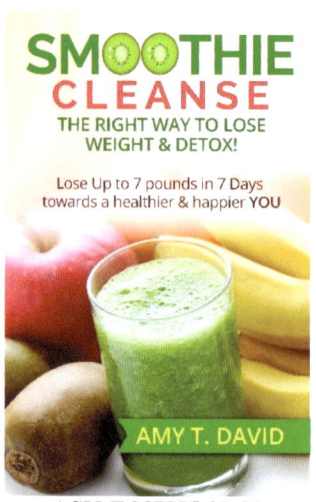

ASN: B00YJO2U88
http://www.amazon.com/dp/B00YJO2U88

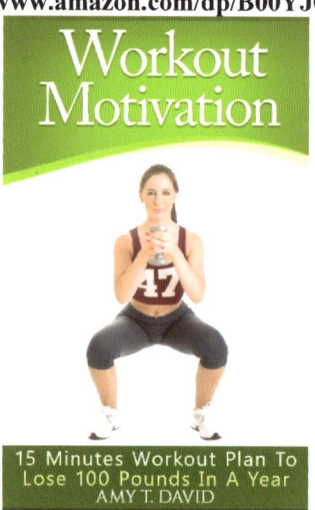

ASIN: B015MHFQCM
http://www.amazon.com/dp/B015MHFQCM